DR SEL  CANCER

Instructional cookbook Manual on How to Treat Cancer

Naturally Using Diet in 2020/2021

Dr Jane A. McCall

Table of Contents

DR SEBI DIET FOR CANCER 1

INTRODUCTION 5

CHAPTER 1 7

    What's Dr. Sebi diet plan? 7

CHAPTER 2 17

    Dr Sebi Meals List: The Very Best Electrical and Alkaline Foods for Your Wellness 17

CHAPTER 3 27

    The Anti-Cancer Diet plan: Foods That Prevent Malignancy 27

CHAPTER 4 38

    Can Turmeric Deal with Prostate Malignancy? 38

CHAPTER 5 49

    13 Foods That Could Decrease Your Threat of Cancer

.... 49

CHAPTER 6 68

12 Beneficial Fruits to consume After and during Cancer Treatment 68

CHAPTER 7 83

Can Alkaline water Treat Cancer? 83

How to make use of alkaline water 83

Risks and warnings 84

Where may I get alkaline water? 84

What can you do now? 85

A c k n o w l e d g m e n t s 86

Copyright © 2021 by Dr Jane A. McCall

All rights reserved. No part of this publication may be reproduced, distributed, or transmitted in any form or by any means, including photocopying, recording, or other electronic or mechanical methods, without the prior written permission of the publisher, except in the case of brief quotations embodied in critical reviews and certain other non-commercial uses permitted by copyright law.

INTRODUCTION

Dr. Sebi was a world-renowned pathologist, herbalist, and naturalist, he left this world in the year 2016, despite the fact, that he is deceased, his discoveries and self-invention on cancer cure are still helping millions of cancer patients around the world During his time on earth. Dr. Sebi healed millions of cancer individuals with his method and his death has done little to change this, he left behind holistic healing for cancer, you can learn from his life and what he believed about this deadly disease to eradicate cancer from the surface of the earth. This vegan diet cleanses the mucus membrane. In doing so, the skin, blood, and lymphatic system get the boost they need to avert cancer disease and every other illness in the body. The popular Usha village that is usually referred to in Dr. Sebi's stories is a tropical healing village with a facility that is dedicated to the growth of Dr. Sebi's vegan diet combination.

CHAPTER 1

What's Dr. Sebi diet plan?

Dr. Sebi thought the Western method of disease to become ineffective. He kept that mucus and acidity - rather bacteria's and viruses, for instance - triggered the disease.

A primary theory behind the dietary plan is that disease can only just endure in acidic environments. The purpose of the diet is usually to accomplish an alkaline condition in the torso to be able to prevent or eradicate the disease.

The diet's official website sells botanical remedies it claims will detoxify your body. A few of these remedies - known as African Bio-mineral Stability health supplements - retail at $1,500 per bundle.

The website links to no research that could support its

statements about health advantages. It does remember that the meals and Medication Administration (FDA) never evaluated the claims. Those behind the website acknowledge they are not medical doctors and don't plan the site's content material to displace medical advice.

How exactly to follow the dietary plan

Dr. Sebi's dietary guide carries several guidelines, such as:

- Just eat foods listed in the guide.
- Drink 1 gallon of organic spring drinking water daily.
- Avoid pet products, crossbreed foods, and alcohol.
- Stay away from a microwave, that may "kill your meal."
- Avoid canned and seedless fruits.

The Dr. Sebi diet plan involves consuming:

- Vegetables, including avocado, kale, bell peppers, and crazy arugula

- Fruits, including apples, bananas, times, and Seville oranges

- Grains, including rye, outrageous grain, and quinoa

- Natural oils, including avocado, hempseed, coconut, and olive natural oils, though the diet plan advises against using the second option two in cooking

- Nuts and seed products, including hemp and uncooked sesame seed products, tahini butter, and walnuts

- Natural teas, including chamomile, fennel, and ginger varieties

- Organic sweeteners, including agave syrup and date sugar

- Spices, including cayenne and powdered seaweed

What are the huge benefits?

There's a lack of any kind of scientific evidence to aid the Dr. Sebi diet plan.

However, research shows a plant-based diet plan can benefit wellness. Some health advantages of plant-based diet programs can include:

Weight reduction - a 2015 research figured a vegan diet plan resulted in more excess weight reduction than other less strict diets. Participants dropped up to 7.5% of body weight after six months on the vegan diet.

Appetite control - a 2016 research in young man participants discovered that they felt more complete and happier after consuming a plant-based meal containing peas and coffee beans when compared to a meal containing meats.

Changing the microbiome - the word "microbiome"

collectively identifies the microorganisms in the gut. A 2019 research discovered that a plant-based diet plan could alter the microbiome favorably, resulting in less threat of disease. Nevertheless, confirming this will demand more research.

Reduced threat of disease - a 2017 review figured a plant-based diet plan may decrease the risk of cardiovascular system disease by 40% and the chance of developing metabolic syndrome and type 2 diabetes by fifty percent.

The Dr. Sebi diet plan encourages visitors to consume entire foods and avoids processed food items. A report from 2017 discovered that reducing the consumption of prepared food would enhance the dietary quality of the overall diet in America.

Is it secure?

The Dr. Sebi diet plan is definitely restrictive, and it

could not consist of enough important nutrition, that your diet's website will not clearly acknowledge.

If a person adopts the dietary plan, they may reap the benefits of consulting a doctor, who might recommend additional products.

Vitamin B-12

Following a Dr. Sebi diet plan may create a supplement B-12 insufficiency. A person might be able to prevent this by eating healthy supplements and fortified foods.

Vitamin B-12 can be an important nutrient essential for the fitness of neural and blood cellular material and to make DNA.

Generally, people following vegan or vegetarian diet plans and older adults have a threat of B-12 deficiency. Doctors generally recommend that people that usually do not consume animal items take B-12 products.

Symptoms of B-12 insufficiency include tiredness, depressive disorder, and tingling in the hands and feet. Gleam threat of pernicious anemia, which will keep your body from generating enough healthy reddish blood cells.

Protein

In the dietary plan, protein helps support the fitness of the brain, muscle tissue, bone fragments, hormones, and DNA.

In accordance with current guidelines, females older than 19 must have a regular protein intake of 46 grams (g), while men from the same age group should consume 56g.

Some foods contained in the Dr. Sebi diet plan contain protein. For instance, 100g of hulled hemp seed products contain 31.56g of protein, as the same amount of walnuts contains 16.67g of protein. For assessment, 100g of oven-roasted chicken white meat consists of 16.79g from the nutrient.

Nevertheless, the Dr. Sebi diet plan restricts other resources of growing protein, such as coffee beans, lentils, and soy. A person would have to consume an unusually massive amount of permitted protein sources to meet up daily requirements.

Research shows that it's important to consume a multitude of herb foods to soak up enough proteins, that are blocks of proteins. This can be hard when following a Dr. Sebi diet plan.

Omega-3 essential fatty acids

Omega-3 essential fatty acids are essential in the different parts of cell membranes. They support:

- Brain, center, and vision health
- Energy
- The disease-fighting capability

The Dr. Sebi diet plan includes plant resources of omega-3s, such as hemp seed products and walnuts.

However, your body more easily absorbs these acids from animal resources. A 2019 research indicates a vegan diet plan includes little or none of the two omega-3 essential fatty acids unless the individual takes a product.

Anyone following Dr. Sebi's diet plan may reap the benefits of acquiring an omega-3 health supplement.

Recipes

Dr. Sebi's tested recipes often contain uncommon elements or his trademarked botanical supplements. Nevertheless, someone who is not purely adhering to the dietary plan could very easily adapt some dishes to make healthy, plant-based foods:

- Dr. Sebi's 'veggie-ful' smoothie. Try departing out the day sugar, because the drink could be fairly sweet enough without it.

- Zucchini breads pancakes. Maple syrup or coconut sugars could replace the time sugar.

- Veggie fajitas tacos. Individuals who consume whole wheat or corn may choose these kinds of tortillas.

CHAPTER 2

Dr Sebi Meals List: The Very Best Electrical and Alkaline Foods for Your Wellness

Dr. Sebi thought that there have been six fundamental meals organizations: live, natural, dead, cross, genetically altered, and drugs.

His diet plan essentially cut out all of the food groupings except live and uncooked, encouraging dieters to consume as close to an organic vegan diet as you possibly can.

This consists of foods like naturally grown fruits & vegetables, as well as whole grains.

Dr. Sebi thought that the natural and live foods had been

"electrical," which fought the acidic meals waste in the torso.

Along with his diet, Dr. Sebi created a summary of foods that he regarded as the very best for his diet plan and called this the Dr. Sebi Electrical Food List.

Actually, after his moving, the Dr. Sebi item list is growing and evolving.

Sticking with the Dr Sebi Diet Plan and Food List could be difficult if you consume out a whole lot. Because of this, you should get accustomed to preparing a whole lot of foods at home.

To greatly help with this, we created a Vegan Meals for the Spirit Cookbook product/game plan that provides you all the information you will need to eat correctly, map out your meals, and also have fun, flavorful quality recipes that abide by the diet.

This way there is no need to put an excessive amount of

thought into everything you need to eat as well as the less thought you must put in the diet, the simpler it'll become to adhere to the diet.

Dr. Sebi Vegetable List

As with almost all his electrical foods, Dr. Sebi kept the fact that people should eat non-GMO foods. This consists of vegetables & fruits which have been produced seedless or modified to contain much more minerals and vitamins than they are doing normally. The Dr. Sebi set of vegetables is quite large and varied, with a lot of options to produce different dynamic foods. This list contains:

- Amaranth
- Arame
- Avocado
- Bell Pepper
- Chayote

- Cherry and Plum Tomato
- Cucumber
- Dandelion Greens
- Dulse
- Garbanzo Beans
- Hijiki
- Izote floral and leaf
- Kale
- Lettuce except for iceberg
- Mushrooms except for Shitake
- Nopales
- Nori
- Okra
- Olives
- Onions

- Purslane Verdolaga
- Squash
- Tomatillo
- Turnip Greens
- Wakame
- Watercress
- Wild Arugula
- Zucchini

Dr. Sebi Fresh fruit List

While the veggie list is decently lengthy, the fruit list is more restricted, and several types of fruits aren't permitted to be consumed while on the Dr. Sebi diet plan. Nevertheless, the list of the fruits continues to offer fans of the dietary plan a diverse group of options. For instance, all types of berries are allowed around the Dr. Sebi meals list except cranberries, which certainly are a manmade fresh fruit. The list also contains:

- Apples
- Bananas
- Berries
- Cantaloupe
- Cherries
- Currants
- Dates
- Figs
- Grapes
- Limes
- Mango
- Melons
- Orange
- Papayas

- Peaches
- Pears
- Plums
- Prickly Pear
- Prunes
- Rasins
- Soft Jelly Coconuts
- Sour soups
- Tamarind

Dr Sebi Meals List Spices and Seasonings

- Achiote
- Basil
- Bay Leaf
- Cayenne
- Cloves

- Dill
- Habanero
- Onion Powder
- Oregano
- Powdered Granulated Seaweed
- Pure Ocean Salt
- Sage
- Savory
- Sweet Basil
- Tarragon
- Thyme
- Alkaline Grains
- Amaranth
- Fonio
- Kamut

- Quinoa
- Rye
- Spelt
- Tef
- Wild Rice
- Alkaline Sugar and Sweeteners
- Date Sugars from dried dates
- 100% Pure Agave Syrup from cactus

Dr Sebi Natural Teas

- Burdock
- Chamomile
- Elderberry
- Fennel
- Ginger
- Red Raspberry

- Tila

Dr. Sebi Plant List

The herb list may be the majority of the limited of Dr. Sebi's meals lists since it is difficult to acquire an herb that has not been altered. An excellent guideline for the natural herbs is to think about ones you can use when they are selected from the backyard (a non-GMO backyard, obviously). A few of the most flexible herbs within the Dr. Sebi Natural herb list consist of:

- Basil
- Dill
- Oregano
- Onion powder
- Real sea salt
- Cayenne

CHAPTER 3

The Anti-Cancer Diet plan: Foods That Prevent Malignancy

An anti-cancer diet plan is an essential strategy you should use to lessen your threat of malignancy. The American Malignancy Society recommends, for instance, that you take in at least five portions of fruits & vegetables daily and consume the right quantity of food to remain at a wholesome weight. Furthermore, researchers have found that one food that prevents malignancy may be a significant part of an anti-cancer diet plan.

Although selecting cancer-fighting foods in the grocery store with mealtime can't guarantee cancer prevention, great choices can help lessen your risk. Examine these anti-cancer diet recommendations:

Eat a lot of vegetables & fruits. Fruits & vegetables are filled with nutrients and vitamins that are believed to reduce the chance of some types of malignancy. Consuming more plant-based foods also offers you little space for foods saturated in sugar. Rather than filling on prepared or sweet foods, eat fruits & vegetables for snack foods. The Mediterranean diet plan provides foods that battle cancer, focusing mainly on plant-based foods, such as vegetables & fruits, whole grains, legumes, and nut products. Individuals who follow the Mediterranean diet plan select cancer-fighting foods like essential olive oil over butter and seafood instead of reddish meat.

Sip green tea extract throughout your daytime. Green tea is a robust antioxidant and could be a significant portion of an anti-cancer diet plan. Green tea extract, a cancer-fighting meal, may be useful in preventing liver organ, breasts, pancreatic, lung, esophageal, pores, and skin cancer. Researchers statement that a non-toxic chemical substance found in green tea extract, epigallocatechin-3 gallate, functions against urokinase (an enzyme important for cancer development). One glass of green tea consists of between 100 and 200 milligrams (mg) of the anti-tumor ingredient.

Eat more tomatoes. The study confirms the antioxidant lycopene, which is within tomatoes could be stronger than beta-carotene, alpha-carotene, and supplement E. Lycopene can be a cancer-fighting meal associated with safety against certain malignancies such as prostate and lung malignancy. Make sure to prepare the tomato vegetables, as this technique produces the lycopene and helps it be accessible to your body.

Use essential olive oil. In Mediterranean countries, this monounsaturated body fat is trusted for both cooking food and salad essential oil and may be considered a cancer-fighting meal. Breast cancer is 50 percent reduced in Mediterranean countries than in America.

Treat on grapes. Reddish grapes have seed products filled up with super antioxidant activin. This cancer-fighting chemical substance, also within burgandy or merlot wine and red-grape juice, may provide significant security against particular types of malignancy, cardiovascular disease, and various other chronic degenerative illnesses.

Use garlic clove and onions abundantly. Analysis has discovered that garlic clove and onions can prevent the forming of nitrosamines, effective carcinogens that focus on several sites in the torso, usually the digestive tract, liver organ, and breasts. Certainly, the greater pungent the garlic clove or onion, the greater abundant the chemically energetic sulfur substances that prevent malignancy.

Eat seafood. Fatty seafood - such as salmon, tuna, and herring - consists of omega-3 essential fatty acids, a kind of fatty acid that is linked to a lower life expectancy threat of prostate malignancy. Unless you currently eat seafood, you may consider adding it to your anti-cancer diet plan. Yet another way to include omega-3s in your daily diet is by consuming flaxseed.

Become proactive, and make more area in what you eat for the next foods that prevent malignancy.

Add Garlic clove to Your Anti-Cancer Diet

Research demonstrates garlic clove is a cancer-fighting meal. Several large researchers have discovered that those who eat even more garlic clove are less inclined to develop types of malignancy, specifically in digestive organs like the esophagus, belly, and colon. Elements in the pungent lights may maintain cancer-causing substances within you from operating, or they could keep malignancy cellular material from multiplying.

Specialists don't understand how much you will need to consume to prevent malignancy, but a clove each day may be useful.

Berries Are Foods That Battle Cancer

As a very tasty deal with and cancer-fighting food, berries are hard to beat. Berries include particularly effective antioxidants, meaning they can halt a normally occurring process in the torso that creates free radicals that may damage your cellular material. Substances in berries also may help maintain cancers from developing or spreading. Therefore, in your anti-cancer diet plan, pick up a small number of blueberries, blackberries, strawberries, or whichever are your preferred out of this large category of healing fruits.

Tomatoes Might Protect Males from Prostate Cancer

Some analysis has discovered that tomatoes can help protect men from prostate malignancy. The juicy reddish-colored fruit might help safeguard the DNA within your cellular material from damage that may lead to malignancy. Tomatoes include a high focus on a highly effective antioxidant known as lycopene. The body may absorb lycopene better from prepared tomato foods such as sauce, meaning whole-wheat pasta with marinara sauce is a delicious method to get your dosage of cancer-fighting foods.

Add Cruciferous Vegetables to Your Anti-Cancer Diet

Cruciferous vegetables - the group containing broccoli, cabbage, and cauliflower - could be particularly useful cancer-fighting foods. Experts have discovered that parts in these vegetables can protect you from the free radicals that harm your cellular material' DNA. They could also protect you from cancer-causing chemical substances, help sluggish the development of tumors, and encourage malignancy cells to pass away. They're a very tasty and healthful addition to your anti-cancer diet plan.

Drink green tea extract to avoid cancer

The leaves from the tea plant (Camellia sinensis) consist of antioxidants known as catechins, which might assist in preventing cancer in many ways, which includes keeping free radicals from damaging cells. Laboratory research has discovered that catechins in tea can reduce tumors and decrease tumor cell development. Some - however, not all - research in humans also has linked consuming tea to a lesser risk of malignancy. Both green and dark teas include catechins, but you'll obtain more antioxidants from green tea extract, so you might want to look at a cup or even more per day inside your anti-cancer diet.

Wholegrains Are in leading Lines Among Foods that Combat Cancer

Based on the American Institute for Cancer Study, whole grains consist of many components that may reduce your risk of malignancy, which includes fiber and antioxidants. A big study including almost half of a million people discovered that consuming more whole grains may lower the chance of colorectal malignancy, making them a high item in the group of foods to combat malignancy. Oatmeal, barley, brownish grain, and whole-wheat breads and pasta are examples of whole grains.

Turmeric Might Reduce Cancer Risk

This orange-colored spice, a staple in Indian curries, contains an ingredient called curcumin (different than cumin) which may be useful in reducing cancer risk. Based on the American Malignancy Culture, curcumin can inhibit some types of malignancy cells in lab studies and slower the spread of malignancy or reduce tumors in a few pets. This cancer-fighting meal is simple to discover in food markets, and you may use it in several recipes on your anti-cancer diet.

Add Leafy Vegetables To Your Anti-Cancer Diet

Leafy vegetables like spinach and lettuce are great resources of the antioxidants beta-carotene and lutein. You'll also discover this nutrition in vegetables that are more typically eaten prepared, like collard greens, mustard greens, and kale. Based on the American Institute for Malignancy Research, some laboratory studies have discovered that chemical substances in these cancer-fighting foods may limit the development of some types of cancer cells.

Grapes Prevent Malignancy from Starting or Spreading

Your skin of red grapes is an especially rich way to obtain an antioxidant known as resveratrol. Grape juice and burgandy or merlot wine also contain this antioxidant. Based on the Nationwide Malignancy Institute, resveratrol could be useful in keeping malignancy from starting or spreading. Laboratory studies have discovered that it limits the growth of several types of malignancy cells.

Cancer-Fighting Beans Might Lessen Your Cancer Risk

Certain fruits & vegetables and additional plant foods obtain a lot of recognition to be good resources of antioxidants, but beans frequently are unfairly overlooked from the picture. Some coffee beans, especially pinto and crimson kidney coffee beans, are outstanding resources of antioxidants and really should be contained in your anti-cancer diet plan. Coffee beans also contain dietary fiber, which might also lessen your threat of cancer, based on the American Cancer Society.

CHAPTER 4

Can Turmeric Deal with Prostate Malignancy?

Prostate malignancy occurs when a malignant cellular material type is in the prostate. The prostate is usually a little, walnut-sized gland between a man's bladder and rectum. About 1 in 5 American males will be identified as having prostate malignancy in his life time.

Researchers have discovered that turmeric and its own extract, curcumin, can help prevent or deal with prostate malignancy. The warm, bitter spice consists of anticancer properties that may quit the spread and development of cancerous cellular material. If you're thinking about using turmeric medicinally, speak to your doctor about any of it. They can examine you to determine whether this is the greatest addition to your present regimen.

The health great things about turmeric

Benefits: Turmeric can be an anti-inflammatory.

The spice's main active component, curcumin, has antibiotic properties.

It's thought to deal with conditions that range from belly ulcers to cardiovascular disease.

Turmeric has wide-ranging health advantages. It's been utilized as an anti-inflammatory treatment in the Chinese language and Indian folk medications for centuries. Some individuals use turmeric to take care of:

- Inflammation
- Indigestion
- Ulcerative colitis
- Stomach ulcers
- Osteoarthritis

- Heart disease

- High cholesterol

- Liver problems

- Viral and bacterial infections

- Wounds

- Neurogenerative diseases, including Parkinson's disease and multiple sclerosis

Researchers in a single 2015 study Supply found that curcumin, which may be the particle behind turmeric's color and flavor, may restrict several cell-signaling pathways. This can be able to prevent or weaken tumor cellular production.

Another study discovered that curcumin may end cancer-associated fibroblasts. Fibroblasts are connective cells that create collagen and additional fibers. These materials may donate to prostate cancer.

It's thought a mix of curcumin and alpha-tomatine, which is situated in tomatoes, might help quit the development of malignancy cells. It could even increase the loss of life of cancer cellular material.

Curcumin also offers radioprotective and radiosensitizing properties. These can help make tumor cellular material more vulnerable to rays while also safeguarding the body against its dangerous results. A 2016 Resource discovered that curcumin supplementation can improve a person's antioxidant position while going through radiotherapy. The analysis determined that can be carried out without harming the therapy's performance.

Researchers within earlier research determined that curcumin supplementation might lessen lower urinary system symptoms connected with radiotherapy.

How to make use of turmeric

The roots from the turmeric plant are boiled, dried out,

and ground right into a good consistency to produce this spice. It's found in everything from meals and textile dye to natural medicine. And a cooking food spice, turmeric can be available as:

- A supplement
- A fluid extracts
- An organic tincture

You should shoot for 500 milligrams (mg) of curcuminoids, or around 1/2 teaspoon of turmeric natural powder, per day. Dosages of just one 1,500 mg of curcuminoids, or around 1-1/2 teaspoons of turmeric natural powder, per day, could cause side effects.

If you don't want to consider it like a supplement, you can even utilize the spice in food preparation. Put in a dash from the spice to your egg salad, sprinkle it on some steamed cauliflower, or blend it into brownish rice. For the greatest results, add dark pepper to the formula. The piperine in the pepper can help your body correctly absorb the curcumin.

You can even enjoy turmeric as a soothing tea. Simmer with each other drinking water and a mixture of the following elements for ten minutes:

- Turmeric
- Cinnamon
- Clove
- Nutmeg

Once you're done simmering, strain the combination and add dairy and a drop of honey for sweetness.

Dangers and warnings

Risks

Turmeric could cause abdominal pain or various other side effects if you ingest huge amounts of it.

If turmeric makes contact with your skin layer, it's

possible to see inflammation.

You shouldn't take turmeric supplements when you have certain conditions or take certain medications.

Turmeric supplements are usually considered safe for many people. When found in moderation, they're typically thought to trigger little-to-no unwanted effects. When used in huge amounts, the degree of its results isn't clear, while some folks have reported stomach discomfort.

Memorial Sloane Kettering warns against acquiring turmeric supplements if you're acquiring particular medications or have specific medical ailments. Turmeric may agitate bile duct blockage, gallstones, and additional gastrointestinal issues, such as stomach ulcers.

The spice could also reduce the ramifications of drugs such as reserpine, which can be used to take care of high blood circulation pressure, as well as anti-inflammatory indomethacin.

You should avoid turmeric if you are using blood thinners, as it might boost your bleeding risk. It's also advisable to avoid turmeric invest in diabetes medication since it can lower bloodstream sugar.

It draws out, curcumin which could cause allergies on your skin, including rash, inflammation, and redness.

Other remedies for prostate cancer

Prostate cancer treatment may alleviate symptoms and improve yourself. Various kinds available treatments consist of:

- Chemotherapy
- Radiation therapy
- Radiopharmaceutical therapy and bisphosphonate therapy for prostate cancer that's spread towards the bone

- Hormone therapy eliminates or blocks bodily hormones and stops malignancy cell growth
- Biologic therapy, which increases, manuals, or restores your body's organic cancer-fighting defenses
- Radical prostatectomy to eliminate the prostate
- Lymphadenectomy to eliminate pelvic lymph nodes
- Surgery to eliminate prostate tissue

Surgery could cause negative effects, for example:

- Impotence
- Urine leakage
- Stool leakage
- Shortening from the penis
- Radiation therapy may also trigger impotency and urinary problems.

Hormone therapy can lead to:

- Sexual dysfunction
- Hot flashes
- Weakened bones.
- Diarrhea
- Itching
- Nausea

Research facilitates incorporating turmeric and its extract, curcumin, into the treatment solution. The spice offers have been shown to lessen the spread of malignancy, as well as prevent precancerous cellular material from getting tumorous. If you intend to add the spice to your routine, remember the next:

- The recommended dosage is 1/2 teaspoon each day.
- You may encounter side effects if you consume

turmeric in larger amounts.

- You shouldn't utilize the spice when you have certain conditions or take certain medications.

You should consult with your doctor about how exactly often and just how much turmeric to use. Although turmeric may possess benefits, no proof suggests using the spice being a standalone treatment choice.

CHAPTER 5

13 Foods That Could Decrease Your Threat of Cancer

All that you eat may drastically affect many areas of your wellbeing, including your threat of developing chronic illnesses like cardiovascular disease, diabetes, and malignancy.

The introduction of cancer, specifically, has been proven to become heavily influenced by your daily diet.

Many foods contain helpful compounds that may help reduce the growth of cancer.

There are also several studies showing a higher intake of particular foods could be related to a lesser risk of the condition.

This guide will explore the research and appearance of 13

foods that may decrease your threat of cancer.

1. Broccoli

Broccoli contains sulforaphane, a grow compound within cruciferous vegetables that might have potent anticancer properties.

One test-tube research showed that sulforaphane reduced the scale and quantity of breast cancer cellular material by up to 75%.

Likewise, animal research discovered that treating mice with sulforaphane helped kill away prostate cancer cells and decreased tumor volume simply by a lot more than 50%.

Some studies also have found that an increased intake of cruciferous vegetables like broccoli could be linked to a lesser threat of colorectal cancer.

One evaluation of 35 research showed that consuming more cruciferous vegetables was connected with a lower threat of colorectal and cancer of the colon.

When you have broccoli with a few foods per week it comes with some cancer-fighting benefits.

However, take into account that the available study hasn't looked straight at how broccoli may affect malignancy in humans.

Instead, it's been limited by test-tube, animal, and observational research that either looked into the consequences of cruciferous vegetables or the consequences of a particular substance in broccoli.

2. Carrots

Several researchers have discovered that consuming more carrots is associated with a decreased threat of particular types of cancer.

For instance, an analysis viewed the outcomes of five research and figured eating carrots might reduce the threat of stomach malignancy by up to 26%.

Another study discovered that an increased intake of carrots was connected with an 18% lower probability of developing prostate malignancy.

One research analyzed the diet programs of just 1,266 individuals with and without lung malignancy. It discovered that current smokers who didn't eat carrots had been 3 times as more likely to develop lung malignancy, compared to those that ate carrots more often than once weekly.

Try incorporating carrots into your daily diet as a wholesome treat or delicious part dish just a couple of times weekly to improve your intake and potentially lessen your risk of malignancy.

Still, understand that these studies also show an association between carrot consumption and malignancy, but don't take into account other factors that are likely involved.

3. Beans

Beans are saturated in dietary fiber, which some research has found can help drive back colorectal malignancy.

One research followed 1,905 people who have a brief history of colorectal tumors and discovered that those that consumed more cooked, dried coffee beans tended to truly have a decreased threat of tumor recurrence.

Animal research also discovered that nourishing rats black coffee beans or navy coffee beans and inducing cancer of the colon blocked the introduction of malignancy cells by up to 75%.

In accordance with these outcomes, eating several servings of coffee beans every week may boost your fiber intake and help reduce the chance of developing cancer.

However, the existing research is bound to animal research and research that displays association, however, not causation. More research is needed to analyze this in human beings, specifically.

4. Berries

Berries are saturated in anthocyanins, herb pigments that have antioxidant properties and could be connected with a reduced threat of cancer.

In one study, 25 people who have colorectal cancer were treated with bilberry extract for a week, which was found to lessen the growth of cancer cells by 7%.

Another small research gave freeze-dried dark raspberries to individuals with dental cancer and showed it decreased degrees of specific markers connected with cancer progression.

One animal research found that providing rats freeze-dried dark raspberries reduced esophageal tumor occurrence by up to 54% and decreased the number of tumors by up to 62%.

Likewise, another animal research showed that giving

rats a berry extract was found to inhibit several biomarkers of cancer.

Predicated on these findings, which include an offering or two of berries in what you eat every day can help inhibit the introduction of cancer.

Take into account that these are pet and observational research taking a look at the effects of the concentrated dosage of berry removal, and more individual research is necessary.

5. Cinnamon

Cinnamon is famous for its health advantages, including its capability to reduce blood sugars and ease swelling.

Furthermore, some test-tube and animal research has discovered that cinnamon can help block the spread of cancer cells.

A test-tube study discovered that cinnamon draw out could reduce the spread of malignancy cellular material and induce their loss of life.

Another test-tube research showed that cinnamon gas suppressed the development of mind and neck malignancy cells, and in addition significantly reduced tumor size.

Animal research also demonstrated that cinnamon extract induced cell loss of life in tumor cells, and in addition, decreased just how much tumors grew and spread.

Which includes 1/2-1 teaspoon (2-4 grams) of cinnamon in what you eat per day could be beneficial in malignancy prevention and could come with various other benefits as well, such as decreased blood glucose and reduced inflammation.

6. Nuts

Research has discovered that consuming nuts could be associated with a lower threat of certain types of malignancy.

For instance, a report viewed the diet plans of 19,386 people and discovered that eating a larger amount of nut products was connected with a decreased threat of dying from malignancy.

Another research followed 30,708 individuals for 30 years and discovered that consuming nut products regularly was connected with a decreased threat of colorectal, pancreatic, and endometrial malignancies.

Other research has discovered that particular types of nut products may be connected to a lower malignancy risk.

For instance, Brazil nut products are saturated in selenium, which might help drive back lung malignancy in people that have a minimal selenium position.

Likewise, one animal research showed that feeding mice walnuts decreased the growth rate of breast cancer cells simply by 80% and decreased the number of tumors simply by 60%.

These results claim that adding nut products to your daily diet every day may lessen your risk of developing cancer in the foreseeable future.

Still, more research in humans is needed to determine whether nut products are in charge of this association, or whether additional factors are participating.

7. Olive Oil

Olive oil can be loaded with health advantages, so it's simply no wonder it's among the staples of the Mediterranean diet.

Several researchers have even discovered that an increased intake of essential olive oil may help drive back cancer.

One substantial review composed of 19 research showed that folks who consumed the best amount of essential olive oil had a lesser threat of developing breast cancer and malignancy of the digestive tract than people that have the cheapest intake.

Another study viewed the cancer prices in 28 countries all over the world and discovered that areas with an increased intake of essential olive oil had decreased prices of colorectal malignancy.

Swapping away other oils in what you eat for essential olive oil is certainly a straightforward way to benefit from its health advantages. You will be able to drizzle it over salads and prepared vegetables or use it within your marinades for meats, fish, or chicken.

Though these studies also show that there could be a link between essential olive oil intake and cancer, presently there are likely various other factors involved as well. More research is needed to go through the direct ramifications of essential olive oil on malignancy in people.

8. Turmeric

Turmeric is a spice famous for its health-promoting properties. Curcumin, its active component, is a chemical substance with anti-inflammatory, antioxidant as well as anticancer effects.

One study viewed the consequences of curcumin upon 44 sufferers with lesions in the digestive tract that could have grown to be cancerous. After thirty days, 4 grams of curcumin daily decreased the number of lesions present by 40%.

Inside test-tube research, curcumin was also found to diminish the spread of cancer of the colon cells by targeting a particular enzyme linked to cancer growth.

Another test-tube research showed that curcumin helped destroy off mind and neck malignancy cellular material.

Curcumin in addition has been shown to work in slowing the development of lung, breasts, and prostate malignancy cellular material in another test-tube research.

To discover the best outcomes, shoot for at least 1/2-3 teaspoons (1-3 grams) of floor turmeric each day. Use it as a surface spice to include taste in foods, and set it with dark pepper to greatly help increase its absorption.

9. Citrus Fruits

Eating citric fruits such as lemons, limes, grapefruits, and oranges continue to be associated with a lesser risk of malignancy in some research.

One large research found that individuals who ate an increased amount of citric fruits had a lesser threat of developing malignancies from the digestive and top respiratory system tracts.

A review taking a look at 9 studies also discovered that a larger intake of citric fruits was associated with a reduced threat of pancreatic malignancy.

Finally, an assessment of 14 studies showed a high

intake, or at least three portions weekly, of citric fruit, reduced the chance of stomach cancer by 28%.

These studies claim that including several servings of citric fruits in what you eat every week may decrease your threat of developing particular types of cancer.

Take into account that these researches don't take into account other factors which may be involved.

10. Flaxseed

Saturated in fiber as well as heart-healthy fat, flaxseed could be a healthy addition to your daily diet.

Some research shows that it could even help decrease cancer growth and help kill off cancer cells.

In one research, 32 women with breast cancer received the flaxseed muffin daily or a placebo for over per month.

By the end of the analysis, the flaxseed group had decreased degrees of particular markers that measure tumor growth, as well as a rise in cancer cell death.

In another study, 161 men with prostate cancer were treated with flaxseed, which was found to lessen the growth and spread of cancer cells.

Flaxseed is saturated in dietary fiber, which other researchers has found to become protective against colorectal malignancy.

Try adding one tablespoon (10 grams) of floor flaxseed into your daily diet every day by mixing it into smoothies, sprinkling it over cereal and yogurt, or adding it to your preferred baked goods.

11. Tomatoes

Lycopene is a substance found in tomato vegetables that is in charge of its vibrant red colorization as well because of its anti-cancer properties.

Several researchers have discovered that an elevated intake of lycopene and tomatoes may lead to a reduced threat of prostate cancer.

An assessment of 17 research also discovered that a greater intake of natural tomatoes, prepared tomatoes, and lycopene were all connected with a lower risk of prostate cancer.

Another research of 47,365 people discovered that a larger intake of tomato sauce, specifically, was associated with a lower threat of developing prostate cancer.

To help boost your intake, add an offering or two of tomatoes in what you eat each day with the addition of these to sandwiches, salads, sauces, or pasta dishes.

Still, understand that these studies also show there could be an association between eating tomatoes and a lower life expectancy threat of prostate malignancy, however, they don't take into account other factors that may be involved.

12. Garlic

The active component in garlic is allicin, a compound that is proven to kill off cancer cells in multiple test-tube studies.

Several researchers have found a link between garlic intake and a lesser risk of specific types of cancer.

One research of 543,220 individuals found that those that ate plenty of Allium vegetables, such as garlic clove, onions, leeks, and shallots, had a lesser risk of tummy cancer than those that rarely consumed them.

A report of 471 guys showed a higher intake of garlic clove was related to a lower risk of prostate malignancy.

Another study discovered that participants who ate plenty of garlic, as well as fruit, deep yellow vegetables, dark vegetables, and onions, were less inclined to develop colorectal tumors. However, this study didn't isolate the effects of garlic.

Predicated on these findings, which includes 2-5 grams

(approximately one clove) of new garlic into your daily diet each day might help you benefit from its health-promoting properties.

However, regardless of the promising outcomes showing an association between garlic and a lower risk of cancer, more studies are required to examine whether other factors be involved.

13. Fatty Fish

Some research shows that including several portions of fish in what you eat every week may lessen your threat of cancer.

One large research showed a higher intake of seafood was connected with a lower threat of digestive tract malignancy.

Another research that followed 478,040 adults discovered that eating more seafood decreased the chance of developing colorectal malignancy, while reddish and processed meats improved the chance.

Specifically, fatty fish like salmon, mackerel, and anchovies contain essential nutrients such as vitamin D and omega-3 essential fatty acids which have been linked to a lesser risk of cancer.

For instance, having adequate degrees of vitamin D is thought to drive back and decrease the risk of malignancy.

Furthermore, omega-3 essential fatty acids are believed to block the introduction of the condition.

Shoot for two portions of fatty seafood per week to obtain a hearty dosage of omega-3 essential fatty acids and supplement D, and also to maximize the health benefits of those nutrients.

CHAPTER 6

12 Beneficial Fruits to consume After and during Cancer Treatment

There's no key that your daily diet makes a difference in your threat of developing cancer.

Similarly, filling on well-balanced meals is important if you're being treated for or dealing with cancer.

Particular foods, including fruits, contain health-promoting substances that may sluggish tumor growth and reduce particular unwanted effects of treatment to greatly help ease your street to recovery.

Listed below are the 12 greatest fruits to consume after and during cancer treatment.

Fruit options for those with malignancy

When becoming treated for or dealing with cancer, food choices are extremely important.

Cancer remedies like chemotherapy and rays could cause many unwanted effects, which may be possibly worsened or improved with what you take in and drink.

Common unwanted effects of chemotherapy and radiation include:

- Fatigue
- Anemia
- Nausea
- Vomiting
- Adjustments in appetite
- Diarrhea
- Constipation
- Painful swallowing
- Dry mouth

- Mouth sores

- Impaired focus

- Mood changes

Filling your daily diet with nutritious foods, which includes fruits, assists supply the body with vitamins, minerals, and antioxidants during your cancer treatment.

However, it's vital that you tailor your fresh fruit choices to your unique symptoms.

For instance, puréed fruits or fresh fruit smoothies certainly are a good option in case you have difficulty swallowing, while fruits full of fiber will help promote regularity in case you are experiencing constipation.

You may even want to prevent certain fruits depending on your symptoms. Such as, citrus fruits may irritate mouth sores and worsen the sensation of dry mouth.

Lastly, entire fruits like apples, apricots, and pears are hard for people with cancer to consume because of mouth sores, difficulty swallowing, dry mouth, or nausea.

1. Blueberries

Blueberries certainly are a nutritional powerhouse, packaging plenty of dietary fiber, supplement C, and manganese into each providing.

They're also abundant in antioxidants and also have been well studied for his or her cancer-fighting results.

Blueberries also may help alleviate chemo mind, a term used to spell out problems with memory space and focus that some individuals experience during malignancy treatment and recovery.

One small research found that consuming blueberry juice daily for 12 several weeks improved storage and learning in older adults.

Similarly, a recently available overview of 11 studies reported that blueberries improved several areas of brain function in children and adults.

2. Oranges

Oranges certainly are a common kind of citric fruit, favored because of their sweet flavor, vibrant color, and stellar nutritional profile.

Just one moderate orange can fulfill and exceed your daily requirements for vitamin C, almost all while supplying additional important nutrition like thiamine, folate, and potassium.

Vitamin C performs a key part in immunity and may help strengthen your disease-fighting capability after and during malignancy treatment.

Research shows that supplement C may decrease the growth and spread of cancer cells and become therapeutic against certain types of cancer.

Supplement C from oranges may also raise the absorption of iron from foods. This can help drive back anemia, a common side-effect of chemotherapy

3. Bananas

Bananas could be a great nutritional addition for all those recovering from malignancy.

They're not merely simple to tolerate for all those with swallowing troubles but also an excellent supply of much important nutrients, including supplement B6, manganese, and supplement C.

Additionally, bananas include a kind of fiber called pectin, which may be especially good for those experiencing diarrhea due to cancer treatments.

Because bananas are abundant in potassium, they can also help replenish electrolytes dropped through diarrhea or throwing up.

Furthermore, test-tube research possesses observed that pectin can help drive back the development and advancement of cancer of the colon cells.

Having said that, more research is required to determine

if the pectin within bananas could slow malignancy cell development in humans.

4. Grapefruit

Grapefruit is a nutritious fresh fruit packed with antioxidants, nutritional vitamins, and minerals.

Furthermore, to provide a hearty dosage of vitamin C, provitamin A, and potassium, it's abundant with beneficial substances like lycopene.

Lycopene is a carotenoid with potent anticancer properties. Some study suggests that it could reduce certain unfavorable unwanted effects of malignancy treatments, such as chemotherapy and rays.

One research in 24 adults discovered that consuming 17 oz. (500 ml) of juice from citric fruits, which includes grapefruit, increased blood circulation to the mind, which could help mitigate chemo brain.

Take into account that grapefruit might hinder certain

medications, therefore it's better to speak to your doctor before adding it to your daily diet

5. Apples

Apples aren't only one of the very most popular fruits but also probably one of the most nutritious.

Each offering is abundant with fiber, potassium, and vitamin C - which can benefit malignancy recovery.

The fiber within apples can promote regularity and keep things moving through your digestive system.

Potassium impacts your fluid stability and can assist in preventing water retention, a common side-effect of some types of chemotherapy.

Finally, vitamin C functions as an antioxidant to aid immune function and fight cancer cell growth

6. Lemons

Known for his or her sour flavor and signature citrus

scent, lemons deliver a burst of vitamins, minerals, and antioxidants.

They're saturated in supplement C, but also contain some potassium, iron, and supplement B6.

Test-tube studies have discovered that lemon extract can help prevent the development of various kinds of cancer cellular material.

Some animal studies show that one compound in lemons, including limonene, could increase your feeling and fight stress to combat depression and anxiety.

While more analysis is required to confirm these findings in human beings, enjoying lemons in your preferred drinks and desserts as a part of a healthy diet plan could be beneficial.

7. Pomegranates

Pomegranates are delicious, nutritious, and filled with health benefits, producing them an excellent addition to any diet plan.

Like various other fruits, they're saturated in vitamin C and dietary fiber but also pack a lot of vitamin K, folate, and potassium.

Plus, some study has discovered that consuming pomegranates might improve your memory space, that could help those suffering from impairments in concentrate or concentration due to chemotherapy.

A report in 28 people showed that consuming 8 oz. (237 ml) of pomegranate juice daily for four weeks resulted in increased brain activity and improved memory.

What's more, pet studies have discovered that pomegranates can help decrease joint discomfort, another common side-effect of cancer remedies like chemotherapy.

8. Mulberries

Mulberries certainly are a kind of colorful fresh fruit

from the same family with figs and breadfruit.

They have already been used to take care of cancer in lots of traditional types of medicine, and emerging research has begun to verify their potential cancer-fighting results.

Mulberries are mostly of the fruits abundant with both supplement C and iron, which might help drive back anemia due to cancer treatments.

They've also saturated in a kind of flower fiber referred to as lignins, which were proven to enhance defense function and kill cancer cells in test-tube studies.

Extra studies needed to evaluate if eating mulberries in regular amounts could be beneficial after and during cancer treatment.

9. Pears

Pears are versatile, filled with taste, and easy to take pleasure from within a healthy diet plan.

They're also extremely nutritious, offering a wealth of

dietary fiber, copper, supplement C, and supplement K in each provision.

Copper, specifically, performs a central function in defense function and minimizes your body's susceptibility to contamination, which may be beneficial during malignancy treatment.

Like additional fruits, pears may contain effective cancer-fighting compounds.

A report in over 478,000 people demonstrated a higher intake of apples and pears was connected with a lower threat of developing lung cancer.

Anthocyanins, a kind of vegetable pigment within pears, are also associated with decreased cancer development and tumor development in test-tube studies

10. Strawberries

Because of their fresh, fairly sweet taste, strawberries certainly are a favorite among fresh fruit lovers.

They are abundant with vitamin C, folate, manganese, and potassium, along with antioxidant compounds like pelargonidin.

Furthermore, to boasting an extraordinary nutritional profile, strawberries might offer many perks specific to malignancy recovery.

First, ripe strawberries are soft, producing them ideal for those with moderate swallowing difficulties.

What's more, one pet study demonstrated that administering freeze-dried strawberries to hamsters with oral cancer helped reduce tumor formation.

Another research in mice discovered that strawberry extract helped eliminate breast malignancy cells and prevent tumor growth.

11. Cherries

Cherries certainly are a type of rock fruit that is one of the same genus as peaches, plums, and apricots.

Each offering of cherries gives a hearty dosage of vitamin C, potassium, and copper.

These little fruits will also be a good way to obtain antioxidants like beta carotene, lutein, and zeaxanthin, which can benefit your wellbeing.

Many reports have discovered that the antioxidants within cherries may help slow the growth of cancer cells.

For instance, one test-tube research showed that cherry extract killed and stopped the spread of breast cancer cellular material.

Another animal research observed comparable findings, noting that one compound present in tart cherries reduced the growth of colon cancer cells in mice.

However, these researchers analyzed the consequences of highly focused cherry extracts. Extra research is required to evaluate if these results also connect with human beings when cherries are consumed in normal quantities.

12. Blackberries

Blackberries certainly are a kind of berry significant for their nice, yet slightly bitter flavor and deep crimson hue.

This popular fruit is saturated in vitamin C, manganese, and vitamin K.

Blackberries also contain a range of antioxidants, including ellagic acidity, gallic acidity, and chlorogenic acidity.

According to some analysis, eating berries can help drive back DNA harm, neutralize harmful substances called free radicals, and gradually the growth and spread of cancer cells.

Additional test-tube and pet studies claim that blackberries may preserve brain health insurance and enhance storage, potentially preventing specific unwanted effects of chemotherapy.

CHAPTER 7

Can Alkaline water Treat Cancer?

Alkaline water is thought to help counteract the acidity that's within your bloodstream. Some theorize that any tumor cells found in the body will starve because cancer cells thrive within an acidic environment.

However, alkaline water won't result in a significant change, under normal circumstances. The body has multiple, complicated, and interrelated mobile mechanisms involved in maintaining your internal pH where it ought to be.

How to make use of alkaline water

If you'd prefer to use alkaline water, you may be in a position to leverage it as your regular plain tap water.

But, maintain in mind that an excessive amount of alkaline water could cause side effects, such as upset belly and indigestion.

Risks and warnings

Normal water with a well-balanced pH is essential. It could have a negative impact on your health. Your body isn't made to drink alkaline water alone. If you drink an excessive amount of alkaline water, this can lead to indigestion or abdomen ulcers.

Your body could also have a problem digesting and absorbing nutrition. Speak to your doctor before making use of it as it might be harmful.

Where may I get alkaline water?

Bottled alkaline water can be available at most food markets. Due to this, alkaline water typically isn't included in your health insurance carrier.

What can you do now?

Although alkaline water is normally considered safe to beverage, If you do opt to give alkaline drinking water a try, here are some tips:

- Once metabolized, adding a press of lime or lemon to your drinking water can decrease the alkalinity because these citric fruits are acidic.

- If you opt to create your alkaline water, use distilled drinking water. This might reduce the number of additives.

- Drinking alkaline drinking water with meals may adversely affect your body's digestive function.

Acknowledgments

The Glory of this book success goes to God Almighty and my beautiful Family, Fans, Readers & well-wishers, Customers, and Friends for their endless support and encouragement.

CPSIA information can be obtained
at www.ICGtesting.com
Printed in the USA
LVHW041034290123
738169LV00014B/284